Anti-Age
This Way
Not That Way

A science-based anti-aging plan that remarkably slow down and reverse your age.

Kristine Knutson M.D

Kristine Knutson

Anti-Age This Way Not That Way

Treat your skin gently

Eat a healthy diet

A healthy diet can help you look and feel your best. Eat plenty of fruits, vegetables, whole grains and lean proteins. The association between diet and acne isn't clear — but research suggests that a diet rich in vitamin C and low in fats and carbohydrates may promote younger looking skin.

Dealing with Wrinkles

Fibroblast

Age Spots

Making Your Skin Younger

Anti-Age This Way Not That Way

`

INTRODUCTION

WHAT MAKES THE DIFFERENCE

People are different and that makes all the difference when it comes to aging even among identical twins.

The biggest factor that influence this difference is *choice*. What people choose to do and not do?

Hardly anyone looks their age.

Most look way older than their real age and research shows that this is true for 80 percent of people.

If you will look older or younger depends on one thing – YOU!

You decide your cellular age like your destiny. Will you act on life or wait for life to act on you? Aging depends majorly on your logic to life.

Are you *reactive* or *proactive*? If you are *proactive* you will look younger and stay younger. The opposite is true for being *reactive*.

If you learn the big secret in this book, you would look younger and feel younger because you are younger literally (because that's what happened to your cells).

You would have the skin, vitality, energy and mental acuity as proofs.

Anti-Age This Way Not That Way

Why do some 70 year olds look 40, running marathons, giving speeches, autographing their bestselling books, living a productive, active life while their counterpart can't even use the loo without assistance not to mention suffering dementia, diabetes and heart diseases?

What makes the former something everyone wants and the latter what no one wish for.

Was that just *chance* or *good genes*?

According to research, our genes only influence 20 -30 percent of how we look as we age this is true even among identical twins, the other factors are due to factors within our influence

Celebrities are quite an interesting bunch. The allure of going under the knife to grab the promise of looking younger is one thing that most times don't work out as hoped.

Many celebrities look terrible after surgery, they look worse off frankly.

Most didn't feel comfortable under their skin and it even got worse when they went for a facelift. The mirror reminds them the pain is still there.

Most people don't need surgery if they truly want to feel and look younger.

You need something that is scientifically based to make you younger for longer, something at the granular level where your cells are actually agile and young not old and sick.

The Peak Look
When kids start talking and making sense of the world, they begin to nurse a desire to grow up fast and join the ranks of grownups.

They see some of the freedoms grownups enjoy not to mention the height advantage.

When people hit a certain age, a new desire to stay young and not to grow old is intense even if some won't admit it.

This book takes you through the steps of how aging works and how to slow and even reverse it.

Aging is a collision race against death and we all know there is something unfair about death. Regardless of how we have come to accept death as part of life, we still feel a tingling sense that death is unfair and unnatural.

Aging is a complex ongoing event that happens to all living organisms.

The normal bodily functions begins to be susceptible to daily wear and tear. The result can be a decline in physical and sometimes mental performance.

But there is good news! A lot of good news!

Anti-Age This Way Not That Way

Recent works on aging has seen unprecedented advances providing us opportunity to expand the health span for longer.

The health span is the number of years you feel healthy as you age. Science has found the ways we can be younger by learning how we could control and even reverse our biological clock.

Kristine Knutson

CHAPTER ONE

YOUR BODY IS MADE OF CELLS

Your body is made of cells just like a house is made of bricks.

How many bricks does it take to make a 300 feet skyscraper?

We will need a lot of bricks for that.

The assembly of the *small* makes the *big* possible. It's the same principle for making long words, the smallest parts to make words, long and short are letters, and we have 26 of such to work with.

With the combinations of letters we can make sentences and then paragraphs, pages and then books.

If we want to make a human size figure on the beach with grains of sand, how many grains of sand do we need to assemble a 6 feet tall human like figure?

Are you thinking about the number?

What quantity comes to mind?

Some sources say between 5 and 10 billion grains of sand.

Kristine Knutson

Well, all living things are made from little round bricks called cells, only that they look different and much smaller than the sand grains we know.

The cell is the building blocks of life. The cell is a lot smaller than a grain of sand.

We can't see our cells with the human eye unless we used an instrument called a microscope, but we can see grains of sand because they are far bigger compared to our cells.

We are composed of trillions of cells. Your hand alone has about 2.5 billion cells, if every cell in your hand was the size of a grain of sand, your hand would be as big as a school bus!

The picture below shows how the cell looks with some organelles (the different parts inside a cell with different functions).

The line is pointing to where the DNA is inside the cell.

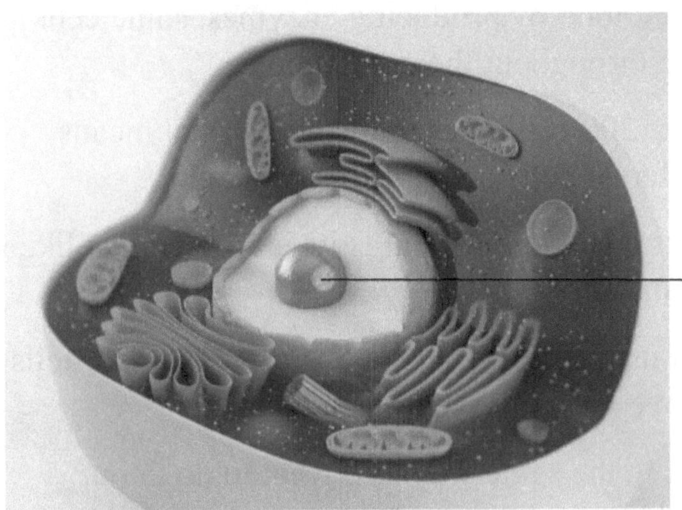

Explaining DNA

DNA is the acronym for deoxyribonucleic acid and is one of the two types of nucleic acid found inside our cells. The other is called RNA, ribonucleic acid.

DNA as stated earlier is a nucleic acid, which has strings of *nucleotides* fused together as well as a backbone made of *phosphate* and *deoxyribose*

DNA is an exquisitely intricate molecule that works in a complex way to control the cell.

Each cell has its own specific job, same way it is with humans.

Some cells enable us perceive light and see, other cells aid us to hear, some cells help us touch, other cells assist us in digesting food by producing enzymes, some cells carry oxygen throughout the entire body.

We have over 200 cell types in the body - that means over 200 different cells doing different jobs!

But how does a cell know what is its job? Well just like it is with humans.

Someone let us know. Just like a boss or supervisor tells a new employee what job to do in a company.

Our cells are in the same way told what to do in our body, but not by a computer or a person this time!

That "telling" job is done by a very special molecule called DNA. So we are back to the DNA again.

DNA—Life's Instruction Manual
DNA is a set of instructions that tells the cell what to become. One way to think of the DNA is to picture it like a set of blueprints for the cell, or say a set of computer codes that tells a PC what to do.

The DNA instruction is written in a unique alphabet that's just four letters long!

Which is unlike a book or computer codes which is 2-Dimensional, and mostly boring – The DNA is a 3-Dimensional curved ladder.

Anti-Age This Way Not That Way

The shape is called a double helix.

Like the ladder, with rungs and handrail, the letters of the DNA alphabet (known as the bases) are the rungs, while special sugars, (deoxyribose) and other atoms, (phosphates) formed the handrail.

The rungs are precisely distinct with a unique name, but they are preferably identified by their initials: A, T, C and G.

Each one pairs up with another like a tag team friend. They are extremely picky about who they tag with.

The alphabet rungs on both sides of the ladder will only pair up in a certain way - just like a jigsaw puzzle.

A and T are one tag team and always pair together

Same goes for G and C, they hang out together every time

Another way to think of it is to visualise A, T, G and C like jigsaw pieces. A and T locks into each other, C and G fit together. Only the right puzzle piece can fit into place, anything different will never work.

Kristine Knutson

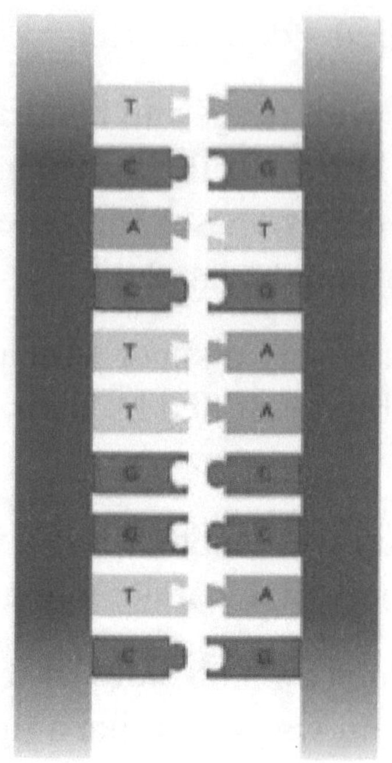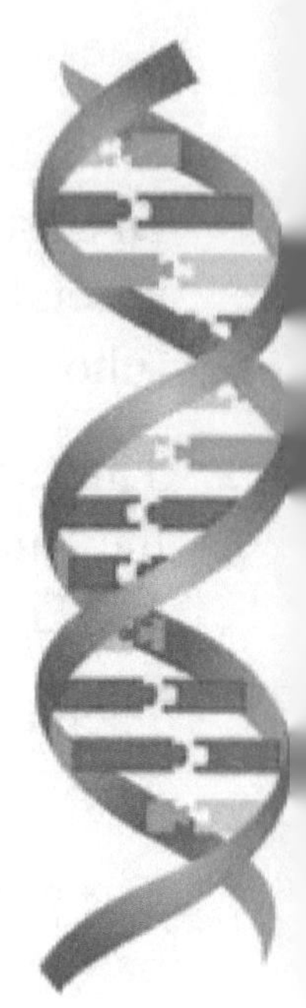

Four Letter Alphabet

Like humans have 26 letters to choose from in making words, so it is with the DNA, it has only 4 letters to combine words with, and each word it combines must be three letters long, known as codons.

If you look at a length of DNA, it appears like this below

ATGCGTGGTCAGTCGATATATGGCCCC

But when you remember they are three letters long, then this is how it should look below

ATG CGT GGT CAG TCG ATA TAT GGC CCC

These are like words that make up sentences that the cell understands. These sentences are akin to what is called genes.

[ATG CGT GGT CAG] [TCG ATA TAT GGC CCC]

Each sentence or gene instructs a cell to produce a peculiar molecule - a protein. It is proteins like these that control everything in a cell.

As an analogy, the DNA can be compared to a boss of a company. It gives out instructions, but much of the actual work is done by others.

It is these proteins that aid each cell to do its job. Each gene (that is, each sentence) makes only one protein.

The Magic of Four Letters
How can four letters give rise to something as intricate as a human body?

If you hand a child 100 pieces of yellow colored Lego pieces to build a tower, despite the child's best efforts, they can only get a yellow colored tower.

But if that child now has a box of Lego with 25 lots of 4 different colours to erect a tower.

Every time they make a tower, they will always have a different combination of colours even when the size of tower remains the same, the colour mix reflected on the tower is different every time the child makes a tower, and we can say the possible combinations is a lot

You should recall it's the sequence of letters that stores the information (just like the order of colors in this analogy).

A set of 3 letters makes a word. From four different letters, we get 64 possible three-letter-words. Can you tell the combinations of words that can result from a sentence of 100 letters?

CHAPTER TWO

TWO TYPES OF AGING

We have learned that the human body is made of small round mini grains called cells.

What happens in our cells affects everything in the human being including how we age.

There are two types of aging for every person. The first is your chronological age, or the number of years you have lived since birth.

The second is your biological or cellular age, this is your age at the level of your cells after putting some factors into consideration like diet, sleep, exercise, heart heath to name a few.

Your biological age also has other names – heart age, functional age or physiological age.

Studies show that most people have an older biological age than their physical age, this is true for 80 percent of people.

The difference between these two aging system explains why some 70 year olds look 40 and are agile, while their counterpart are bed-ridden and sick.

Scientists have studied why these differences persist between two people with similar genetic endowments.

They were able to take a good look at the cellular processes that influence these differences leading to the term "hallmarks of aging"

There are nine provisional hallmarks that signify aging in different organisms, with particular interest on aging in mammals.

These hallmarks are:

1. Genomic instability,
2. Telomere attrition,
3. Epigenetic alterations,
4. Loss of proteostasis,
5. Deregulated nutrient sensing,
6. Mitochondrial dysfunction,
7. Cellular senescence,
8. Stem cell exhaustion, and
9. Altered intercellular communication.

I. Genomic instability

The word *genomic* is from the word *genome*. It is good you have a firm grasp of what a *genome* is and how it is different from an *epigenome*.

The human **genome** is the entire collection of DNA (deoxyribonucleic acid), and this is about 3 billion base pairs - that distinguish one individual from another.

DNA contains the instructions for making the proteins that do most of the work in a cell.

The **epigenome** is an assembly of chemical compounds that direct the **genome on** what to do.

The **epigenome** is used for regulating gene development, expression, tissue differentiation, and suppression of transposable elements.

Unlike the primary **genome**, which is more or less largely static within an individual, the **epigenome** can be largely altered by environmental factors

There are some things that can affect your genome and that could influence how you age, things like exposure to chemicals, smoke or other toxic agents over a long period from the environment leading to simple DNA replication errors or oxidative stress.

Although humans have a multipart network of DNA repair systems, DNA damage mount up over the long haul of our lives, and that triggers mutations in cells, some people may come down with cancer as a result.

II. Telomere attrition

Just like in plastic tips of shoelaces enclosing and protecting their braided ends, telomeres protect the extreme ends of our chromosomes against deterioration.

The regular DNA replication process in most cells are not capable of copying the ends of our DNA completely, and that means the telomere region shortens continuously from each cell division with each repetitive DNA sequencing.

After multiple replications, there is a condition that result called cell growth arrest, restricting the ability of tissues to regenerate as before due to aging.

III. Epigenetic alterations

Have you ever wondered how different tissues and organs come about from the same genetic information stored in every cell?

This is where epigenome goes to work. Epigenetic information tells a cell what tissue or organ to become by (suppressing or expressing) turning off or turning on some genes as necessity demands.

For example, if a cell should end up as a kidney cell, epigenetic modifications will only turn on the parts of the genome specific for kidney cells while turning off other parts specific for other cells.

The aging mechanism alters our epigenetic code in some ways, leading to how genes are expressed differently from what it used to be affecting normal cellular function.

As an example, in the immune system, the balance between turning on and turning off immune cells can be shifted unfavourably, leading to our bodies becoming more susceptible to pathogens.

IV. Loss of proteostasis

In our cells, proteins are frequently being produced and disintegrated, and this activity is identified as proteostasis or protein homeostasis. Proteins are comparable to tools manufactured correctly to perform the multipart cellular functions within each cell.

One part of making proteins correctly is how they are folded into the appropriate shapes.

Various mechanisms have evolved to better stabilize or restore correctly folded proteins, and to remove and degrade improperly shaped proteins which could otherwise accumulate and damage the cell.

When these mechanisms become less efficient over time, damaged or aggregated protein components cause dysfunction or even cell toxicity, as seen in diseases like Alzheimer's.

V. Deregulated nutrient sensing

Cells behave differently when nutrients are in abundant supply and when it is scarce, in abundance, cells and tissues store energy and grow, when there's scarcity, the cells go into protection mode (homeostasis) and do a lot of repair in cells and tissues.

Patients with diabetes and obesity, have cells that are desensitized to such behaviour because there's always abundance in nutrients.

There's a semblance of this happening in aging as cells do not respond as expected to regulate the cell.

VI. Mitochondrial dysfunction

High amount of Free radicals, (known as reactive oxygen species, ROS), generated as a by-product of energy production from mitochondria is damaging to the cell leading to what is known as mitochondrial dysfunction, the more ROS, the more damage it causes in addition to cellular deterioration.

This condition affects different cellular processes negatively, the cell produce less energy, and oxidative stress escalates.

In this way, mitochondrial dysfunction play a part in different age-related disorders such as myopathies and neuropathies.

VII. Cellular Senescence

The combination of DNA damage, telomere shortening and a lot of stress to a cell lead to a state of growth arrest known as cellular senescence.

Cells with this arrest due to genomic damage in some ways prevent the occurrence of cancer at the expense of that cell not being able to replenish itself.

Senescent cells behave differently from their prior functions, they start secreting harmful molecules into the cell environment.

These pro-inflammatory secretion leads to a range of geriatric issues among which are kidney dysfunction and osteoarthritis.

VIII. Stem cell exhaustion

One observation that comes with oldage is the slow recovery to injury, this is due to decreased ability of the stem cells to replace damaged tissues.

These stems are dormant most of the time but when they are triggered to repair tissues and wounds, their effectiveness is hindered by DNA damage, cellular senescence and telomere shortening, with time this leads to a condition called stem cell exhaustion

IX. Altered intercellular communication

For a cell to work optimally and grow, it must send and receive messages with other cells through signalling molecules.

Cells or tissues can transmit messages via the blood stream using molecular messengers to cells/tissues far away.

Aging affects signals sent and ability of cells to respond to these signals efficiently.

This communication dysfunction is responsible for problems like chronic tissue inflammation, in addition to immune system failure to identify and clear out pathogens or dysfunctional cells, increasing vulnerability to infection and cancer.

These are the characteristics that explains aging, we have to learn what speeds up aging and slows it down.

Anti-Age This Way Not That Way

CHAPTER THREE

THE THINGS THAT SPEED UP AGING

There's actually a DNA clock in our bodies that tells how old we are, this information can be verified by an expert checking your blood sample.

They will be looking for chemical groups that get added and subtracted to your DNA, as you age.

Everyone gets chemical modifications in predictable ways as one gets older starting from conception, so even in the womb even as a kid even as a teenager you're aging based on this clock that goes up linearly and will you fit on that line, it's very accurate in telling your biological age.

Some experts can go as far as predicting how long you would live base on the information on this clock.

We call it the Horvath clock by measuring these little chemicals that accumulate on the DNA like a plaque on the teeth

Methylation is when chemicals like hydrogen and oxygen bound to the DNA chemically, and those accumulate as you get older in very predictable ways in fact they're so predictable that the same clock can tell the dog's age as well as a human's age

There are two classes of enzymes, the ones that add the methyl chemicals and those that subtract them, many scientist believe when they learn how to induce enzymes to take away the methyl chemicals then that action holds a promise for age reset or age reversal if you like.

Some of the agents that make people age really fast is exposure to radiation from a number of sources like the Sun as well as x-rays and CT scans unless if your doctor says go for it please don't refuse that but otherwise don't do it for fun or curiosity because those CT scans breaks your DNA.

For example, when a mouse DNA is broken, its age goes up by 50% so you want to avoid situations that breaks your DNA as much as possible

Ionizing radiation is high-energy radiation… it's got a lot of energy. When this high-energy particle or wave hits an atom, the atom absorbs the energy; causing the weakest electron to pop off! This creates a charged atom called an ion!

Do that enough and all that high-energy can cause chemical changes in our cells and tissue.

If ionizing radiation affects too many cells at once, or we absorb a bunch over time -- that's when we risk sickness, radiation poisoning, or eventually cancer.

That happens when the radiation changes how things fit together. It might knock off bits of our DNA, mess with its structure, or (at worst) break one or both strands of the DNA double helix!

The way that cell stress causes aging

One other way people age really fast is due to cell stress, it is when cells lose their packaging ability and then eventually lose their identity and they become zombie-like and then senescence sets in and that may even leads to organs failure.

The packaging ability of a cell is the really important part because much like the software runs the code in a computer to perform a specific task or set of tasks, the same way the epigenome controls which genes are turned on and off,

But all that change if there is stress to the system and by that I mean biological stress and the biggest stress for a cell is to break its chromosome that event is a major setback and it's really harmful to the body, like there could be a tumor.

For such emergency, the cell gets to work, it stops some other activity to concentrate on the crisis at hand, it does two things, it stops dividing and then tries to repair that broken DNA by recruiting proteins from somewhere else that's already doing a good job of making sure the cell's functioning correctly, those proteins are used by the cell to repair the DNA that's broken

When a DNA is broken, one can't fix it or glue it unless it is first unpacked and then stick back together and afterwards repack it, so this movement of proteins and the unpacking and repacking of the DNA might just be the reason cells lose their original youthful agility

So DNA breakage is bad enough, but the unpacking and repacking as a result of that adds to the problem of aging.

I must add that it is safe to keep your smartphone away from your bedroom while you are ready to retire for the night.

What proteins are and how they work

Proteins are actually little machines like we said, they run the activities that takes place in a cell.

They create chemical reactions that normally would take a billion years to happen this is what an enzyme does that accelerates reactions and so we've got about 20,000 different types of enzymes in the body and they do different things

What's really exciting in the last 20 years is we've discovered that one can make those proteins responsible for packaging and repairing the DNA correctly very efficient by doing the following

- exercise
- dieting
- intermittent fasting

These are some ways these enzymes that control our body mechanisms make us healthier by making those enzymes much more active and efficient, keeping you younger for longer

CHAPTER FOUR

THE THINGS THAT SLOW DOWN OR REVERSE AGING

Hypothesis vs. Hypothesis

In the middle of the last century, the hypothesis was that it was damage to our DNA, mutations to our DNA that happened over the course of our lives that makes us get older but, recent evidence has suggested that that is not really the case.

I mean, you can take an adult cell, and you can clone it into a new organism. And that organism appears to live about as long as non-cloned organisms of the same species.

So in that way it seems like all the information is still there in the DNA. So if we're not losing information in our DNA then what is the reason for aging?

Well, recent studies appears to point to the loss of information, but not the information in our DNA, in our genome but the loss of information in in our epigenome. So what is the epigenome?

Every cell in your body has the same DNA, but, different cell types have different epigenomes.

They have different ways of packaging that DNA, coiling up, so that it's not read, and leaving some parts of the DNA spooled out, so it's easier to transcribe and turn into proteins and run that cell.

So the epigenome is responsible for turning on or turning off different parts of the DNA.

The way it does that is with proteins called 'histones' that, essentially, the DNA is wrapped on, and also things like methylation.

So there's these chemical signaling markers which are placed on the DNA in certain positions.

So the idea is: when your body is first forming, the epigenome is what tells your cells what type of cell to become. But as you get older, it appears they are losing some information in the epigenome.

And that's important because if a skin cell needs to remain a skin cell, it's up to the epigenome.

And if you don't have the epigenome the skin cell will forget what type of cell it is and it might turn into another cell.

You start to get hair growing where it shouldn't: ears, nose, and back. That's cells losing their identity, the cells go:

"I can't remember what I'm supposed to do, I'm not reading the right genes anymore."

Anti-Age This Way Not That Way

So, the key to this sort of breakdown in the epigenome is DNA damage.

Yeah, so when you go out in the sun, or be exposed to CT scan and X-ray or some other type of radiation, you'll break your chromosomes.

And in the effort that the cells go to stick the chromosome back together, note: the DNA isn't just flailing around, it's actually bundled up.

The cell has to unwrap it, recruit proteins to help, join it together, and then they have to go back and reset the structures.

And that resetting of the epigenome happens about 99%. The loss of 1% in efficiency is the aging process.

So overtime, histones are not returned to the right places and DNA methylation is added in places where it shouldn't be.

Your Longevity Genes

Humans like bacteria have 'longevity genes'. These genes triggered by adversity create enzymes which among other things, maintain the epigenome

We have these 'hormetic response' genes or 'longevity genes' that are in all of our cells, and they sense

- when we've run a lot,
- we've lost our breath or

- we're hungry,
- we are a little bit hot,
- or a little bit cold.

These genes turn on our general defences against aging.

So, what is that? So, when parts of our cells fall apart: they can put them back together. Proteins misfold: they can get rid of them or put them back together.

The ends of the chromosomes get shorter: they can lengthen them. A lot of processes that go on but one of the most important, I think, is maintaining the information, the epigenetic information in the cell, so that our cells don't forget what to do or become..

There are three types of longevity gene. There are the ones we work on called 'sirtuins' and they control the information in the cell.

In fact, 'sir' in sirtuins stands for 'silent information regulator' number two (SIR2).

There are other ones. The other group is called AMP-kinase or AMPK. This group of genes senses how much energy we're taking in... Mostly in the form of sugar.

And then the third group is called mTOR. And these genes control and respond to how much amino acids we're taking in.

We don't want to eat too much meat as this will prevent mTOR from helping you live longer.

Anti-Age This Way Not That Way

And so, a molecule called 'NMN', raises the level of a chemical called 'NAD', in the cell that makes it stimulate hyperactive defences in the body.

So to sum up, there are six things that you can do right now to slow the rate of your aging.

Number one: avoid DNA damage. Wear sunscreen, avoid x-rays and all sort of harmful radiation.

Number two: eat less. Caloric restriction.

Number three: eat less protein, because your body has ways of detecting how much of that you're taking in.

Number four: do some exercise. 'High-intensity interval training' (HIIT).

Get your heart rate up to 85%, make your body feel like you're running from a lion or from some danger.

Number five: be uncomfortably cold, or (there is still ongoing research how this can be safely performed).

Number six: be uncomfortably hot (there is still ongoing research how this can be done to maximise the benefit).

All of these things will trigger your body's 'longevity genes' into maintaining your epigenome.

Going into 'repair and protect mode' rather than 'grow and reproduce', and if you think about those things, those are generally all the things that we don't do.

Reversing aging

Here is what some research on reversing aging suggest.

Back in 2012, a scientist named *Yamanaka* received the Nobel Prize for discovering four factors, which when applied in a gene therapy to an adult cell, would reset the whole epigenome back to how that cell was when it was an embryo.

So it is called 'pluripotent stem cell'.

Now, you wouldn't want to apply that to your entire body because, well, then you would turn into a giant tumor because your cells wouldn't know how to differentiate.

But it does suggest that there are ways of resetting your epigenome, and they could be the key to reversing aging.

From the works of *Yamanaka,* a mouse almost going blind was restored to clear vision by using just three of the four reprogramming factors that won the Nobel Prize.

One factor was left out called 'cMyc', which causes cancer, and the other three seem to be just the right recipe for taking the age of the eye backwards, but not too far to stem cell status.

So the big question is: if there was success in reversing the cells in the eyes of a mouse, can it work the whole body of the mouse so it becomes totally younger?

Anti-Age This Way Not That Way

Well, there is an ongoing research on that but success in the eye therapy gives scientist some hope.

Age reset was possible for the eye tissue in mice but it is still not possible for an entire human body yet.

So in order for this to actually work and reset an entire human body, we would need another way, and this is where the jellyfish come in, because 'moon jellyfish'— any cell in an adult jellyfish can actually be reset into an earlier stage of its life cycle.

It can become a polyp again. So it seems like the jellyfish are actually capable of activating something like the Yamanaka factors and resetting their epigenomes to an earlier time in their lives.

If we were able to figure out how they do that, well, then maybe we could do the same with our own cells.

We do have the ability to reset our epigenomes, but that is typically only used when we're in the embryonic stage, when we need to maintain all our cells as stem cells.

As we age, most mammals including humans, lose stem cells over time.

And the stem cells we do have become more and more restricted over time to the types of cells they can make.

So if we can understand how the 'moon jellyfish' can take, presumably, many different kinds of cells, and reverse-engineer them into the cells it needs during regeneration, which might give us an idea of how to do it in ourselves, as well.

So, we're still some way off from reversing aging in the entire human body. But there's at least a roadmap.

Anti-Age This Way Not That Way

CHAPTER FIVE

THE SKIN

The skin is a reflection of the several factors that influence aging, from radiation to diet, stress to sleep, exercise to intermittent fasting.

Your skin is what keeps score on how well or worse you are aging.

Your skin, the largest organ in your body, protects inner tissues and organs from the outside environment.

It's essential to take good care of the skin so it will help you stay healthy as you age.

Unfortunately, a skin that has lost its youthful glow can be a concern.

A certain study found that people looked five years younger when skin discoloration was removed from their photos.

And a digital smoothing of wrinkles lopped off a whopping 15 years. But, how can you get young, fresh-looking skin?

Your diet and lifestyle play a major role in how your skin looks. For younger, fresher looking skin, you want to cut back on sugar and refined carbs.

Anti-Age This Way Not That Way

Anything that is sugar or gets rapidly converted to sugar could attach to collagen and cause stiffness of skin and very old looking skin.

Drinking water regularly to keep you hydrated is one habit that will keep you fresh looking throughout the day.

Nothing keeps your skin hydrated and supple better than drinking water regularly.
You want to indulge generously in fruits and veggies.

A diet rich in fruits and vegetables will provide you with plenty of antioxidants that will help protect your skin and overall health.

Good skin care, including sun protection and gentle cleansing can keep your skin healthy and glowing for years to come.

Don't have time for intensive skin care? Pamper yourself with the basics.

Good skin care and healthy lifestyle choices can help delay the natural aging process and prevent many skin problems.

Get started with these five no-nonsense tips.

Protect yourself from the sun

Exposure to cold temperatures or too much sun can cause premature wrinkles and dry, irritated skin

Kristine Knutson

One of the most important way to take care of your skin is to protect it from the sun.

A lifetime of sun exposure can cause wrinkles, freckles, age spots and rough, dry skin.

Sun exposure can also cause more-serious problems, such as skin cancer. For the most complete sun protection:

Avoid the sun between 10 a.m. and 4 p.m. This is when the sun's rays are the strongest.

Wear protective clothing. Cover your skin with tightly woven long-sleeved shirts, long pants and wide-brimmed hats. You might also opt for special sun-protective clothing, which is specifically designed to block ultraviolet rays while keeping you cool and comfortable.

Use sunscreen when you're in the sun. Apply generous amounts of broad-spectrum sunscreen 30 minutes before going outdoors and re-apply every two hours, after heavy sweating or after being in water.

Smoking

Smoking makes your skin look older and contributes to wrinkles. Smoking narrows the tiny blood vessels in the outermost layers of skin, which decreases blood flow.

This depletes the skin of oxygen and nutrients, such as vitamin A, that are important to skin health. Smoking also damages collagen and elastin — fibers that give your skin its strength and elasticity.

In addition, the repetitive facial expressions you make when smoking — such as pursing your lips when inhaling and squinting your eyes to keep out smoke — may contribute to wrinkles.

If you smoke, the best way to protect your skin is to quit. Ask your doctor for tips or treatments to help you stop smoking.

Quitting sticky bad habits is more of a psychological thing than a medical one.

Treat your skin gently

Daily cleansing and shaving can take a toll on your skin, so keep it gentle. Lay off the harsh soaps and cleansers.

Commercial soaps that contain chemicals can dry and irritate your skin.

Limit bath time. Hot water and long showers or baths remove oils from your skin. Limit your bath or shower time, and use warm — rather than hot — water.

Avoid strong soaps. Strong soaps can strip oil from your skin. Instead, choose mild cleansers.

Shave carefully. To protect and lubricate your skin, apply

shaving cream, lotion or gel before shaving. For the closest shave, use a clean, sharp razor. Shave in the direction the hair grows, not against it.

Pat dry. After washing or bathing, gently pat or blot your skin dry with a towel so that some moisture remains on your skin.

Moisturize dry skin. Find a moisturizer that fits your skin type and makes your skin look and feel soft.

Eat a healthy diet
A healthy diet can help you look and feel your best. Eat plenty of fruits, vegetables, whole grains and lean proteins.

The association between diet and acne isn't clear — but research suggests that a diet rich in vitamin C and low in fats and carbohydrates may promote younger looking skin.

You want to supplement your diet by taking alpha lipoic acid, Alpha lipoic acid is 400 times stronger than vitamins C and E, and it helps improve your skin by bringing down inflammation.

Take the antioxidant CoQ10, It slows downs the aging process.

Dealing with Wrinkles

People not only fear wrinkles but when they finally appear, people hate dealing with wrinkles.

They see it as a reminder of the impending fear every living being must face.

You should know that the first main cause of wrinkles is the loss of collagen and elastin.

Like the clothes you use, the skin falls victim to the normal wear-and-tear.

When different toxins get on your skin, you may break out. When you are still at the prime of your youth, the skin is able to repair itself easily.

But as you get older, you will notice that scars no longer disappear quickly.

You see the appearance of gaps and holes on your skin. The two important proteins in your body, collagen and elastin, are used to repair the skin so that you can prevent fine lines and wrinkles from forming.

When you go past the age of 30, your body won't be able to quickly reproduce collagen and elastin. This means that your skin is on its way to showing its wrinkles.

It also means you need to assist your body system in your daily choices and lifestyle.

Another reason for aging is the loss of hyaluronic acid.

This is a substance that gives the skin cells volume because it is able to retain a certain amount of moisture in the cells.

The larger the cell volume, the less wrinkles you have.

Without this acid, your skin would look dull and dehydrated. Unfortunately, enzymes in the body destroy the acid found in the skin.

Once it is gone, everything else starts to fall apart and you have to face dealing with wrinkles.

Of course, you also have to consider free radicals. This is also one of the main cause of aging.

Free radicals are basically unstable molecules that must stabilize themselves by stealing electrons from other molecules. The more they steal, the more you replicate them. This creates a ripple effect that affects everything else in your skin.

Some women become complacent when it comes to aging and dealing with wrinkles.

Though they don't try to resist it and calmly accept it as a part of life, they also don't do anything about it.

Few explore the "whys" and the "hows" of aging.

Anti-Age This Way Not That Way

Yes, they buy over-the-counter creams.

But do they really understand how these work?

When it comes to your skin, it is only right that you are careful with what you put on it.

Fibroblast

Dermatologists have done research on how you heal. They discovered this small cell called a fibroblast.

Aside from its healing properties, they also found that it can stimulate the production of collagen.

To reverse the effects of aging, you need to spark the production of fibroblasts.

If you can do this successfully, you can rejuvenate your skin back to a more youthful time.

Where can you find medicine that help stimulate the production of fibroblast?

Though most of the good ones are not available on shelves at your local pharmacy or department store, you can talk to your dermatologist about it.

They may be able to give you the proper prescription.

Moreover, you should not do anything to your body without first getting the approval of your doctor. You can be certain that they will know the best options to take with dealing with wrinkles.

Age Spots

Many of us are unhappy with our skin and want to get rid of age spots that don't look attractive at all and sometimes may indicate that we age. But in order to get rid of age spots, first we have to understand how they get on the skin.

As a way to protect itself from the sun's harmful UV rays, your skin releases a dark pigment called melanin.

This is what gets you darker over an extended period under the sun.

Because your body has ways to protect itself, the melanin released sort of acts as a shield to help to protect the tender skin underneath.

If this didn't happen, the inner layer of your skin will suffer irreversible damage because it does not have a way of protecting itself from radiation.

However, this does not give you a free pass to stay under the sun for as long as you want.

Anti-Age This Way Not That Way

When cells become overly damaged, hyper-pigmentation takes place.

You'll know when this happens because you will see dark spots on your skin start to appear.

There is a cure for these unwanted spots, which most people like to refer to as age spots. They do not have to be permanent as long as you utilize products with the right ingredients. You just don't put anything on your skin.

In fact, choosing the right medication must be done with utmost care.

What you need to stay away from is using products that employ the use of chemical agents. Removing age spots the natural way is still the best remedy.

Dermatologists are often asked what they think works best when it comes to get rid of age spots. Answers may differ with every person.

What works for one may not work for the other.

You have to consider your skin type, your health, and your history.

That is why different types of remedies were made so that everybody gets a chance to help their skin look young. Just as a means of information, here are a few of what people use:

This form of topical ointment is applied directly on dark spot to lighten the skin. The best ones out in the market use natural substances as their active ingredients. Look for names such as alpha arbutin and alpha hydroxyl: these are the most effective natural ingredients.

Please avoid chemicals that pose as dark spot remover, chemical peels have acid in them to help remove the outer layers of skin.

When skin peels, the dark spots are removed as well. Some spots may take a few sessions and if you happen to have sensitive skin, you may notice irritation in some areas.

Laser resurfacing is similar to a chemical peel. It also removes the outer layers of skin.

If you want faster results, be willing to shell out some money.

Make sure that you buy makeup or sunblock that contains zinc oxide.

Get a deep cleansing mask, an olive oil daily cleanser, a daytime moisturizer, and an anti-aging night cream to make sure that the whole process can yield faster results.

Cleansing, toning, and moisturizing: *the three most important routines* that help get rid of age spots.

Anti-Age This Way Not That Way

If you make sure that you do this every day, you will see your skin become smoother and look younger in 7 days or less.

Remember, your skin is your body's primary form of clothing, and you will never be able to feel confident if your recklessness and irresponsibility have made you forget to take care of yourself.

When you get rid of age spots you will take care of the largest organ of your body - your skin!

Making Your Skin Younger

A younger looking skin was always a dream of every man and woman. Unfortunately, we all have to face the fact that we will get older.

If your skin is starting to look old, it means that your body isn't as well equipped to deal with the harsh changes.

Your main goal now is to rebuild these defences so that your skin is more able to handle the stress. The word tougher has a lot of connotations, but it does not necessarily have to be negative. People often think of an old piece of leather, and we all know that this is not what we want.

Toughening up your skin means that you have to reactivate your skin's natural ability to treat and repair itself so that you will always look healthy and have a younger looking skin.

You can strengthen your outward appearance and finally feel beautiful.

To start with, when your skin cells are healthy, they are able to produce a lot of structural proteins like collagen and elastin.

These two substances can perform miracles on your skin. They are directly responsible for keeping your skin soft, smooth, and firm.

When you age, your cells aren't as capable in producing these natural substances.

Years of exposure to sunlight and environmental toxins can damage your body's natural ability to repair the areas that have been exposed to harmful substances.

If you happen to read a lot of magazines and watch a lot of TV, you will realize that many cosmetic companies would have you believe in the power of creams and lotions.

However, these aren't always enough. Their highly synthetic chemical ingredients simply act as fillers for your fine lines and wrinkles.

The truth is, these cosmetic tricks only last as long as the next wash.

Anti-Age This Way Not That Way

In order for your skin to be better prepared so that you will look young and fresh, you need the time-tested methods of protection to get your cells back up and running again.

First, you need to avoid regular exposure to sunlight. Be sure to constantly wash away the unhealthy substances with water. Then, you also need to consider your diet.

You need to add more fruits and vegetables to your meals so that you pump up your antioxidant volume.

Say goodbye to radicals because you now have given your body the weapon it needs to fight them. When you have the right amount of nutrients, you will notice a significant improvement in your health.

Proven methods of support continue to prove themselves as the better option. After all, what good is Botox when you still lead an unhealthy lifestyle?

Aside from diet and exercise, you also can supplement your efforts with homemade treatments.

You can use *buttermilk* and *lemon essential oils*. These two substances are known to remove age spots. Combining them will give you better skin, and you don't need to wait long to see the results.

Just mix three drops of lemon essential oil with one tablespoon of buttermilk before you dab it on the different areas of your face. Another effective home treatment is to use sandalwood paste.

Just mix sandalwood powder, lemon juice, cucumber juice and tomato juice to make a paste. Apply this on your skin and let it dry. Wash the gook off with lukewarm water afterwards.

Knowing how to make skin tougher without looking older is a simple matter of giving your skin the proper protection. Love yourself and know that you need to take care of what you have before it's too late your beautiful younger looking skin.

CHAPTER SIX

SLEEP

You look in the mirror in the morning and discover that you have big black circles beneath your eyes, and your energy level is low.

It is hard to think straight. You may be experiencing a medical condition referred to as sleep deprivation.

This problem is brought on by lack of sleep and can badly affect your brain and your body.

Due to some reasons, some people suffer from lack of sleep where they cannot sleep for more than a couple of hours, or they do not sleep for more than a couple of hours because of their schedule.

Some may not know it, but there are ten surprising effects of sleep loss:

- Sleepiness causes accidents
- Sleep loss dumbs you down
- Sleep deprivation can lead to serious health problems
- Lack of sleep kills sex drive
- Sleepiness is depressing
- Lack of sleep ages your skin
- Sleepiness makes you forgetful

- Losing sleep can make you gain weight
- Sleep deprivation engenders the chances of death
- Sleep loss impairs judgment,

Studies show that people who are getting six hours of sleep over time instead of seven or eight begin to feel that they've adapted to that sleep deprivation – they've gotten used to it. But, in their tests of mental alertness and performance, they continue to go downhill.

So, there comes a time in sleep deprivation when we can't grasp how impaired we are.

Caffeine works well in keeping people awake for a short time, but it doesn't work for longer duration.

Health care professionals suggest taking stimulants or short naps or combining both to combat sleep deprivation, but getting more sleep is the only natural cure.

Remember, we covered telomere length in earlier sections of this book.

Did you know that sleep has a lot to do with your telomere length?

It does. Sleep has been associated with a lot of things that should drive health and longevity.

Chronic sleep loss has been associated with Alzheimer's, cancer, diabetes.

Anti-Age This Way Not That Way

In fact, with diabetes, you have a terrible night of sleep, and you have insulin resistance the next two days.

And guess what that might be? Maybe cortisol, depression, immune dysfunction, hypertension all of these things are all associated with chronic sleep loss.

Telomere shortening has also been associated with a shortened lifespan, and sleep loss has been associated with telomere shortening.

Even short-term sleep loss has been associated with decreased gene expressions.

In terms of healthy genes and biomarkers, here's one of the studies. Proceedings of the National Academy of Sciences. "Effects of Insufficient Sleep on Circadian Rhythmicity and Expression Amplitude of the Human Blood Transcriptome." Again, what they're showing is we change the genes that we express based on how well we sleep.

Here's another one. The research from the Whitehall II Cohort Study." What is a telomere anyway?'' discovered that there was a link between short sleep and shorter telomere length in healthy men.

It's the end cap on a chromosome, and it has something to do with the Chroma.

Our body's ability and the chromosome's ability to find specific gene locations pull that gene out and actually translate that gene into RNA and then RNA and proteins, genes, enzymes, things like that.

The shorter your telomere, the shorter your predicted or projected lifespan.

Here's another one in Oxford Sleep. "Association between Snoring and Leukocyte Telomere Length." This research here connects snoring with the telomere length.

Snoring is one thing many of us don't realize we do when we're asleep. Many people have sleep-disordered breathing - sleep apnea.

You may notice that you wake up in the middle of sleep, but you don't notice what woke you up quite often. It was snoring or sleep apnea, or sleep-disordered breathing.

Being interrupted during sleep by the above is detrimental to your health.

When your body is trying to reconstruct and restore hormone levels for carrying out essential work within your body (like lower cortisol levels), continue to get interrupted with sleep disorders, and you continue to hurt your health.

Whatever you do, don't assume you are okay going by with less sleep. Get age reset by practicing healthy sleep that spans 8 hours.

Anti-Age This Way Not That Way

Research shows that men who only sleep 4-5 hours will have a level of testosterone which is that of someone ten years their senior.

So poor sleep will age a man by a ten years in terms of that essential area of wellness. And we see equivalent dysfunction in female reproductive health caused by sleep shortage.

There is a connection between sleep loss and your immune system, and you know there is a link between your immune system and aging.

Your immune system has cells called natural killer cells, and you can think of natural killer cells almost like the secret service agents of your immune system.

They are efficient at spotting dangerous, foreign elements and eliminating them. What they're doing here is destroying a cancerous tumor mass.

So what you want is a valiant pack of these immune terminator at all times, and tragically, that's what you don't have if you're not sleeping enough.

So in an investigation, you won't be sleep-deprived for a whole night, your sleep will be restricted to four hours for one single night, and we would check the percentage of decline in immune cell activity that you got.

And it's not tiny -- it's not 10 percent, it's not 20 percent. The drop in natural killer cell activity was in the 70-percent range.

That's a concerning state of immune deficiency. You can perhaps understand why we're now finding significant links between short sleep duration and your risk for developing numerous forms of cancer.

Currently, that list includes cancer of the bowel, cancer of the prostate, and breast cancer.

The relationship between a lack of sleep and cancer is so significant that the World Health Organization has categorized any night time shift work as a possible carcinogen because of an interruption of your sleep-wake rhythms.

So you may have heard of the advice that you can sleep when you're dead. Without mincing words -- it is mortally deadly advice.

We have reached the conclusion based on epidemiological research across millions of persons. The point is this: shorter sleep leads to shorter life. Short sleep predicts all-cause mortality.

And if increasing your risk for the development of cancer or even Alzheimer's disease were not sufficiently disquieting, we have since discovered that a lack of sleep will even tear down the very building blocks of life itself, your DNA genetic code.

Anti-Age This Way Not That Way

So in a particular study, they assemble a group of healthy adults, and they restricted them to six hours of sleep a night for seven days.

Then they measured the new occurrences in their gene activity profile comparative to when those same persons were having a total of eight hours of sleep at night.

And there were two critical findings. First, a substantial and crucial 711 genes were affected in their activity, due to a lack of sleep.

The second result was that about half of those genes were increased in their activity.

The other half were decreased. Now the affected genes that were turned off by a lack of sleep were genes associated with your immune system, so once again, you can see that immune deficiency.

In contrast, those genes that were up-regulated or increased by way of a lack of sleep were genes connected with the promotion of tumors, genes associated with long-term chronic inflammation within the body, and genes associated with stress, and, as a consequence cardiovascular disease.

Every aspect of your wellness that suffers from sleep deprivation experiences dire results.

Sleep loss will cost every fiber of your physiology, even interfering with the very DNA nucleic alphabet that keeps the cells of your body running.

And at this point, you may be thinking, what do I do differently? What are your tips for good sleep?"

Well, you want to make sure you avoid alcohol and caffeine, avoid naps during the day, and pay attention to these two pieces of recommendations. The first is regularity.

Go to bed simultaneously, wake up at the same time, no matter whether it's the weekday or the weekend.

Regularity is the name of the game, and it will improve the quality and quantity and of your sleep. The second point is temperature.

Your body has to drop its average temperature by, say, two to three degrees Fahrenheit to induce sleep and then to stay asleep, and it's the reason it's hard to fall asleep in a room that's too cold or too hot.

Setting your bedroom temperature at about 65 degrees or around 18 degrees Celsius is advisable; that should be satisfactory for most people.

Sleep is a non-negotiable biological necessity, not an optional lifestyle luxury. It is Mother Nature's life-support system.

Anti-Age This Way Not That Way

And the demolition of sleep in industrialized nations is creating a tragic impact on our wellness, health, safety, and children.

CHAPTER SEVEN

EXERCISE

Exercise are physical actions a person engages to enhance or keep up one's fitness and overall health.

It is performed for varied reasons, including strengthening muscles and the cardiovascular system, honing athletic skills, weight loss or maintenance, and enjoyment.

Researchers have also found that exercise can get deep into your body, even into your DNA.

Accordingly, people who exercise have younger DNA by up to 9 or more years. Indeed, that is an incredible benefit!

That means that keeping fit by exercising can do more than help prevent illness; it may make you younger.

Why exercise?
For individuals wanting to look and feel younger, anti-aging is not only about buying anti-aging products.

Anti-aging is about making the healthiest of choices.

Exercise can prove to be better for the body and, thus, better for anti-aging than any bottled product.

Anti-Age This Way Not That Way

Lack of exercise goes hand in hand with aging. Inactivity leads to the loss of muscle tone and strength.

Your posture and muscles will deteriorate over time due to lack of activity and may cause the skin to sag resulting in that aged look.

Taking the time to care for your body through a regular exercise schedule will prevent the effects of aging from a cellular level.

The benefits of exercise have been shown in study after study. The secret to anti-aging and exercise is just that simple and just that easy to carry through.

Benefits of Pilates Reformer
If you're like most people, you can experience the health benefits of Pilates. These programs do have not only fantastic health benefits but also increase self-confidence and wellbeing.

So, how exactly did Pilates start? During World War I, there was a host of wounded soldiers in need of medical attention.

Many of these wounded soldiers didn't always get the most needed treatment because they were in a chaotic surrounding. Then came a man named Joseph Pilates.

He was a nurse of the German army. He was way ahead of his time because he was able to think of devising a particular form of exercise to address the injury concerns.

What Joseph did was carry out his innovation by attaching weighted springs to the beds of the wounded.

True enough, the patients got well and recuperate faster with the help of this rough device. It was the birth of the first Pilate's equipment from which devised other forms of related tools.

Today, countless physical therapists, chiropractors, osteopaths, and trainers use the rehab exercise program. This rehab program has been shown to help improve a patient's posture, flexibility, and balance.

All in all, exercise strengthens the body. Good form is emphasized in the scheme. You can gain strength in weak and affected muscles. The exercises and movements focus on the joints.

There is a boost of smaller muscle groups supporting the joints and bony structures.

An awareness of balance is then established because the various muscle areas can gain equal strength.

The exercise is no longer dedicated to only those suffering from injuries.

As the health benefits of Pilate exercises are gaining momentum, the exercise has gained popularity in recent years among the general population.

Pilate's instructors incorporate a few tools so that you can participate in the excellent exercise of Pilates.

Anti-Age This Way Not That Way

You can tone and strengthen specific parts of the body if you do it regularly.

You don't need to worry about spending on expensive equipment.

Aside from time, you need to invest in a yoga mat and a couple of comfortable exercise outfits.

If you want to invest in equipment to challenge yourself more, you could get a Pilates ball and some resistance tools.

Pilates helps strengthen the core of your body. It helps to improve the muscles in your stomach, back, and rear end.

If you work on just these three areas, you will see a significant improvement in your entire body.

You will be a lot steadier when sitting, standing, and walking. Besides, you will get better posture due to strengthened core muscles.

Once you have your core strengthened, you will find it more comfortable to sit correctly. Pilate's exercises help lengthen the spine.

You are encouraged to sit and stand properly. If that sounds more like you, you don't need to worry. Doing all these will become easier when you become dedicated to the exercise.

`

Pilates increases your mind-body connection. To successfully perform the exercise, you must set your mind from the very beginning.

Concentrate on your breathing, which is an integral part of Pilates.

Proper breathing demands mental focus unlike other exercise programs. Because Pilates is a low-impact workout, anyone can participate.

Older people do not have to worry about the impact on their sore muscles and joints.

The exercise increases your flexibility while strengthening muscles at the same time. Another benefit of Pilates for women who are overweight is the benefits of Pilate's weight loss.

When you start exercising with Pilates, your body will thank you by making you see the improvement in just a short time. In that short time, the benefits of Pilates come to full fruition, and you'll feel it!

Stretching Exercises
Probably you may have never thought about yoga for anti-aging and that it could be good for your health.

The fascination with eastern mysticism made yoga meditation very popular.

And obviously, stretching your muscles and working on your bones helps you be more flexible and mobile.

Anti-Age This Way Not That Way

Not everybody wants to associate yoga with mysticism and religion but do appreciate a good stretch, so they do yoga just for practical and health reasons, not religion.

Therefore, we do not intend to ponder the goodness of the eastern philosophies and religions, but about the practical part of the little part called yoga exercises.

Those who already train for a while have certainly noticed that they can stretch or even bend their bodies like never before.

Interestingly, the instructors and coaches in yoga exercises can pinpoint your age according to your ability to stretch and bend your body.

Just think about it, the easiness of your body movement can shout your age to others.

Working on your spine in yoga classes will help prevent the degeneration of your skeleton.

It can improve what you have done through the years by feeding your body with a bad diet, abusing your posture by picking up heavy stuff the wrong way, not working, and train your body.

You might be already going down the hill of destruction - if you are not taking care of your body, it will collapse sooner or later.

In a way, your body is like any other machine, and it needs to be maintained.

Now, advertisements in magazines, on television, and on countless billboards invite you to start some diet and join a health club. Let me ask you, why not a yoga class?

Just think how well you will care for your bones and spine by participating in those classes.

Through these kinds of regular exercises, you will improve your general health and bone health.

Naturally, there is a vast difference between people of different ages.

The stretching poses for those who are twenty might look different to those who are fifty years old.

How will the exercises slow down the aging process? Think about what you are going to provide to your body:

- suppleness to your stomach muscles,
- mobility to your spine,
- improving your posture,
- you will remove tensions,
- you will tighten up your skin,
- And remove your double chin.

If you are not in the spring years of your life or have not done any stretch exercises before, talking to your doctor would be the most important thing.

You would need to get the green light from them first. As with other physical activities, you can't start with the most challenging training first.

Anti-Age This Way Not That Way

You will do much better if you start very slowly. Because yoga is like any other training, you must warm up your body to prepare the muscles before you begin.

During the stretching, you might come to the point that you will feel discomfort, especially if you are new to this type of body activity. At this moment, it is advisable to stop and rest.

By following the advice to take it easy and slowly and not overdoing it, you will make steady progress, and you will move to the more complicated phases without any problems.

Remember, it doesn't matter that you did not exercise before. You will get a very flexible body.

Those advanced in years should feel some comfort knowing that studies proved that older people who started doing yoga and fitness have slowed down their aging process and felt more effective than the time before the yoga regime.

Therefore, get ready and get genuinely sincere about slowing down aging using the practice of "asanas."

This particular method calls for deep breathing routines and meditation.

The practice will lead you towards improving and even eliminating digestive disorders, varicose veins, chronic weaknesses, and many other disorders associated with age.

Furthermore, a consistent yoga routine assists you with weight reduction because you will be more conscious of your own body.

You will end up adequately taught to listen and to react to your body's call and needs.

You will discover publications, books, and internet sites that look at your capability to improve your physique further and begin a wholesome alternative lifestyle.

By utilizing yoga exercises, you can expect to live longer simply because you can easily control each of the essential determinants of a long life: brain and mental performance, glands, spine, and internal organs.

Due to the above facts, your entire body will require a lot more oxygen. Each cell in your body is going to be impacted.

Yoga and fitness nourish the cells which might need more oxygen. Now is the time to strengthen your spine and back, enlarge your lung volume, and let yoga be an integral part of your everyday routine to scoop the anti-aging benefits.

Facial Exercises that Keep You Young-Looking
Have you tried facial exercises to prevent wrinkles? No? Then, how long have you been looking for low-cost cream because you either want to prevent new wrinkles or the old ones from disappearing?

You know you're not getting any younger, and the wrinkles are the natural way of becoming old.

Most likely, you are not only afraid of a cosmetic surgeon, but you are not financially capable of affording one.

Right?

I don't want you to despair. Facial exercises are a way to work on your wrinkles, and you'll be happy to hear that it is a cheap method, too.

And, I must say it is perhaps THE BEST organic anti-aging facial care.

Facial exercises will certainly help your skin to look not only healthy but also young-looking.

Don't worry.

The facial exercises are not complicated at all, and you can follow instructions with ease, and they are the cheapest way of anti-aging skincare available.

How to Do Facial Exercises

If you don't know where or how to start, follow few simple steps below, and you certainly will look fresh and younger: There is no trick; there is no magic.

But, it would help if you committed yourself to do the facial exercises every single day.

Then you can be assured that your present wrinkles will begin to smoothen and the potential ones won't form either.

While sitting down straight and looking at the ceiling, chew with your lips closed. Facial Exercises

Keep your lips together and drop your jaw while pushing it forward.

Push your lips forward as far as possible to form an exaggerated "O" with your mouth, and then smile as brightly as you can.

Gently apply pressure to your forehead from the two sides of your temple with your fingers.

Close your eyes and sit upright before you lift your eyebrows and stretch the eyelids down and up to the possible extent.

Frown and lift your eyebrows as far as you can while opening your eyes.

Anti-Age This Way Not That Way

Sit upright, look straight, start bringing your eyebrows down, wrinkle your nose as much as possible, and flare your nostrils.

For those exercises to be practical, you must repeat each one at least ten times. Also, do them for at least 20 minutes.

The goal of those exercises is to affect particular muscles and muscle groups.

The muscle spasms and resistance motion strengthen the facial muscles, and in consequence, your skin will look healthier because of the more excellent blood supply.

As I said before, no tricks and no magic: simple increased blood flow makes your face look fresh thanks to your tighter and more toned skin.

With age, muscles become weaker and flabby. It is very noticeable, especially on your face and neck.

You know that if the muscles around your face and neck sag, you start to look quite old and unattractive not only to yourself in the mirror but to anybody around you.

As you probably care about how you appear to others (and to yourself, too), the flabby look can have a significant impact on your self-confidence.

And the truth is that no tons of makeup or the most fashionable outfit will help cover the lost youth on your visible features, which won't cover the age.

The good news is that the simple methods above will help you to believe in yourself and you'll be able to look in other people's eyes without embarrassment knowing that you look pretty and healthy and young.

And that's thanks to those twenty minutes of your daily activities.

First, when you start getting into daily exercises, you may experience a good feeling of self-consciousness.

True, if you proceed with the facial exercises, you will look "weird" outside onlooker. Therefore, you must carry on with them in the privacy of your room or home.

And for your information, these facial movements are called principal isometric and resistance exercises. As awkward as you may feel while doing them, the daily schedule will significantly affect your face's contour and achieve this with no astronomical cost of cosmetic surgery.

Anti-aging facial exercises help keep everything looking as it did when you were younger. You can tighten the muscles and then let your skin follow suit.

It can mean fewer wrinkles and the disappearance of loose skin.

Anti-Age This Way Not That Way

From the moment you begin this incredible transformation process, you will see the difference every time you perform the movements.

Consider this with just a few minutes of your time each day. You will be able to create visible changes that will turn into long-lasting results.

CHAPTER EIGHT

DIET

Our body is one perfect machine if we learn to just take care of it. If one part of the system stops working properly, the other parts could follow suit.

After all, how can it work well when it cannot deliver the way it was meant to do?

Of all the creatures here on earth, we are supposed to be the smartest of them all. Our brain can do so much if we learn how to use it.

If we just set it to the right frequency, we can adapt habits that will work for our own good. Just like today's well-developed technology, the changes can affect our overall performance.

So how do we take care of our body so that it performs at its optimum levels? The answer lies in the lifestyle we choose.

If we are careless with ourselves, we won't be able to do the many things we were meant for.

What we eat, how we sleep, and how we exercise: all these contribute to how we age.

The old adage "we reap what we sow" can basically sum up how well you will live.

Anti-Age This Way Not That Way

If your diet consists of unhealthy junk, you won't have the energy to do the basic things when you age.

You need the proper nutrition to become active.

As tempting as these foods are, you just cannot survive on empty calories.

If you constantly load yourself up with sweets, fats, and tons of carbohydrates, you will find it somewhat difficult to do anything.

Life has so much to offer you and you need the strength to be able to carry around the extra weight.

Is it so hard to eat healthy?

You may always give in to temptation, but you make up one day to find that you will no longer be allowed to take in almost everything.

Of course, you won't want to live your life tiptoeing around what you can and cannot do. Several older people have actually expressed deep regret with the way they used to live.

If it were only possible to turn back the clock, they'd definitely do things differently.

When you are left with no choice, you will force yourself to learn how to eat healthy foods.

When you just set your mind to it, you can actually learn how to live a healthier lifestyle.

Doctors and experts have been telling you that you need to take care of your mind and body.

Mind goes above everything else because this is the powerhouse of the body.

Give yourself some time to eat well, exercise, and most importantly, rest.

Everything you do has an impact on your brain activity.

Too much junk can deprive you the ability to think straight and live right.

You need to learn the value of sensible eating.

Load yourself with lots of fruits, vegetables, and lean meat. Keep your muscles strong through exercise. You will be able to work much better if you are a little more proactive about your health.

You will be that active older person that every youth looks up to simply because you were able to live right.

Here are some natural foods that will make you look beautiful, younger and healthy. You want to incorporate these foods into your daily meal

Green tea

This natural food is incredible. There are many important healthy elements in green tea, it contains high amount of antioxidants, antioxidants mops off those free radicals that are the by-products of our metabolism.

Anti-Age This Way Not That Way

Free radicals are unstable molecules that steal electrons from neighbouring molecules causing problems in the human body.

Antioxidants neutralises these free radicals, and that's why we need a steady supply of them.

Green tea contains polyphenols which prevent diabetes, insulin resistance and heart disease.

Polyphenols also help us build collagen, which help the skin look smooth and tight not lax and wrinkled. They are also good for our bones.

Dark chocolate

Dark chocolate has a remarkable antioxidant profile that beats other widely talked about foods like cranberries, blueberries and the Asei fruit from Brazil.

This is not the common chocolate you get at the super market.

Dark chocolate is found to reduce blood pressure, arterial function and elasticity, and insulin sensitivity.

They contain flavonoids that protect the skin from sun damage, whether you ingest it or apply directly on your skin, you will reap the maximal benefits – hydration, improved thickness and smoothness.

The magic ingredient in this dark chocolate is cacao, the higher the cacao, the higher the flavonoids. Choose the dark chocolate that has at least 70 percent cacao content.

You can add tiny bit of sugar when taking it.

Spices

There are many spices that should get more credit than they are getting because they not only add flavor to your foods but they also bring healthy benefits and younger skin.

For example, cinnamon helps in the production of collagen, chilli pepper helps against age related changes and ginger brings anti-inflammatory benefits which work against age spots

Bone broth

You can home cook bones from poultry, meat or fish to make a nice bone broth, where you can harvest a lot of collagen leading to a beautiful skin, with increased moisture and elasticity.

A study found out that adding other skin supporting nutrients with collagen for 12 weeks drastically reduce wrinkles in postmenopausal women

Anti-Age This Way Not That Way

Flaxseeds
They have immense health benefits like lower cholesterol, reduce blood pressure and decrease the risk of cancer.

They contain omega-3 acids that protect from sun radiation and Skin damage.

A study conducted shows that women who took flaxseeds oil for 12 weeks had improved hydration and smoothness

They help against sun damage and engender skin quality or smoothness

Vegetables

Every vegetable is one of a kind, when you know how to use them you reap incredible benefits like the prevention of diabetes, heart disease, cataracts and cancer because of the antioxidants they contain.

Many vegetables contains carotenoids which protect against radiations from the sun and free radicals, both hasten skin aging

Other vegetables provide vitamin C, which helps in collagen production not to mention strong antioxidants on the side.

A study shows that taking 180mg of vitamin C daily for 5 weeks improved skin oxidants by 37 percent. That's huge!

There are many more benefits of vegetables, you should add a portion of vegetables to your meal daily

Pomegranates

This fruit may have more antioxidant content than green tea according to some research, they help decrease inflammation, prevent free radicals damage as well high blood trigger levels.

It may also help patients recover quickly from colon cancer.

The fruit helps against skin damage by producing collagen. Do well to consume pomegranate as much as you can.

Extra Virgin Olive oil

This is one of the rarest healthy oil on the planet. It works against blood pressure, metabolic syndrome, cancer and heart disease.

Extra Virgin Olive oil helps make the skin look younger because of the almost 70 percent concentration of mono-saturated fats.

Anti-Age This Way Not That Way

Keep an eye out for a good quality Extra Virgin Olive oil and use daily and reap the benefits in your health and skin

Fatty fish

Fatty fish is one of the healthiest food choice on the earth, they contain rich omega-3 acids, which help against ulcerative colitis, heart disease, skin damage, and inflammation.

Some persons with intense skin damage were given omega-3 for 12 weeks and there was a remarkable improvement on their skin.

The 7 day anti-aging meal plan
Here is a 7 day anti-aging meal plan you can start right now and you will notice a remarkable difference after a week.

1. Remember, the healthiest food choice is the alkaline plant base, when mixed with vegetables, you have a winner. Do well to consume more plant base proteins instead of animal sources.
2. Always stay hydrated daily, take a minimum of 2 litres of water daily.
3. Avoid sugars – glucose, fructose, sucrose, maltose and all their cousins

4. Avoid low-fat foods, they trick people into consuming such foods by using the marketing lingo "low-fat foods". Low fat foods contain high amount of salt or sugar.
5. Drink green tea or white tea instead of caffeine or tea, remember caffeine accumulates in your fatty tissue and causes cellulite production in your body, and you don't want that.

Day One
Breakfast

- Two poached eggs and 6-8 medium size asparagus steamed or one whole grapefruit
- 1 Mug White tea or hot water with lemon and ginger

Mid-Morning

- Palmful of almonds

Lunch

- Lentil and vegetable soup
- 1 big apple
- 1 Mug of green tea

Mid-Afternoon

- Fruit salad

Supper

Anti-Age This Way Not That Way

- Mixed cruciferous vegetable stir fry with coconut milk
- 1 Cup of mung-bean salad with cucumber and 1 tbspn of skin refining dressing
- 1 Mug of chamomile tea

Day Two
Breakfast

- Large skin-enhancing with 1 cup of mixed berries and a small unsweetened yoghurt
- 1 Mug green tea or hot water with lemon

Mid-Morning

- Palmful of walnuts

Lunch

- Salmon
- Spinach and salad with 1 tbspn of skin refining dressing
- Mug fennel tea

Mid-Afternoon

- bean salad

Supper

- Vegetables including chick peas with red-bell peppers and tomatoes with 1 cup cooked wild rice

- 1 Mug of chamomile tea

Day three
Breakfast

- Blueberries and almond milk smoothie
- 1 Mug hot water with ginger

Mid-Morning

- Palmful of almonds

Lunch

- 500ml broccoli and mint soup with 1 slice bread
- 1 Mug of green tea

Mid-Afternoon

- Fruit salad

Supper

- Small organic chicken breast, poached in garlic, onions and marigold vegetable stock powder
- Served with mixed-green vegetables including bean, kale and grated ginger
- 1 Mug of chamomile tea or fennel tea

Day four
Breakfast

- Grapefruit segment from one whole grapefruit with 1 tbsp blanched almonds

Mid-Morning

- Handful mixed pumpkin and sunflower seeds

Lunch

- Salmon fillet served over a whole bag of wilted spinach
- 1 pear
- 1 Mug of white tea

Mid-Afternoon

- Beans salad

Supper

- Leek savoy cabbage, fennel seed and pea
- 1 slice pumper nickle bread
- 1 Mug of fennel tea

Day five
Breakfast

- Bowl of gluten-free porridge, with 1tbsp of chia seeds with almond milk and 50g berries

Mid-Morning

- Palmful of walnuts

Lunch

- Whole avocado, mung-bean sprouts and mixed leaf salad with cooked quinoa and pumpkin seed salad, 1 tbspn of skin refining dressing
- 1 big apple
- 1 Mug of green tea

Mid-Afternoon

- Sardine pate (mash a tin of drained sardine with freshly squeezed lemon juice to taste) and 2 oats cakes

Supper

- Spinach and omelette (made with 2 eggs) with mung-bean sprout and tomato salad and 1 tbsp of skin refining dressing
- 1 Mug of chamomile tea or nettle tea

Day six
Breakfast

- Large slices watermelon with large skin enhancing smoothie

Mid-Morning

- Tahini (sesame seed spread)with 1 oat cake

Lunch

- Mashed avocado, spring onion and crushed tomato

Anti-Age This Way Not That Way

- 1 big apple
- 1 Mug of white tea

Mid-Afternoon

- Almond and spirulina bounce balls

Supper

- 500g of mint and pea soup with 2 tbsp sunflower and pumpkin seeds sprinkled ontop
- 1 Mug of nettle or fennel tea

Day seven
Breakfast

- Skin enhancing with berries
- 1 Mug of hot water with lemon and ginger

Mid-Morning

- Palmful mixed sunflower and pumpkin seeds

Lunch

- Superfood salad (usually a combination of beetroot, beans avocado, chick peas, boiled egg and greens and 1 tbsp of skin-enhancing dressing
- 1 medium pear
- 1 Mug of green tea

Mid-Afternoon

- Tahini with 2 oat cakes

Supper

- Salmon fillet poached in white tea with ginger, garlic and onion served over wilted kale and steamed broccoli
- 1 Mug of chamomile tea

Anti-Age This Way Not That Way

CHAPTER NINE

STRESS

There was a study conducted among 68 identical twins to help identify the factors that contributed to aging. The research provided valuable clues into what makes us look older.

One noticeable discovery was that twins with the same genetic composition age differently from each other. What this means was that the twins age differently in different parts of the body.

Among one twin, one age more in the eyes while the other age more on the jawline.

In another set of twins for example years of sun exposure created much deeper lines for one woman when compared to her sister who spent much less time outdoors

Another important discovery from this study was the big role stress plays between twins. Stress can make one twin to age significantly more than the other, when people are stressed, it takes a big toll on the skin.

The skin becomes uptight and the muscles tighten up and all the blood that is supposed to nourish the skin is shunted and that's how the aging is accelerated.

Anti-Age This Way Not That Way

Stressful life events made one twin look older than the other who obviously had no such hectic life events.

Even when two people share same genes, the difference in their lifestyles make the difference.

Uncontrolled stress can make your skin more sensitive and trigger acne breakouts and other skin problems.

To encourage healthy skin — and a healthy state of mind — takes some steps to manage your stress.

Set reasonable limits, scale back your to-do list and make time to do the things you enjoy. The results may be more dramatic than you expect

Another factor that made a big difference between twins is smoking. A twin that smokes look way older than the non-smoking counterpart.

Fatigue
It's easy to say that you can laugh your way through life just to stay healthy. But when problems come, staying positive can actually be very challenging.

In fact for some, this could even be next to impossible.

Numerous studies reveal that your health can be affected by how you react to stress and anxiety.

In the same way, changing how you see things and being more positive about it can help you live longer and better.

Life is just sweeter when you always see the glass as half-full.

Experts have been saying that the mind and body are closely linked with each other.

If you are constantly depressed and down in the dumps, you usually end up taking your health for granted.

Fact is, it is not the stress itself that gets to you. It's what you do to yourself when you feel the pressure that destroys you.

Negativity is what you must avoid as much as you can if you want to live a full and healthy life.

Constantly feeling low can lead to a number of medical problems. Among which are anxiety, depression, high blood pressure, headache, ulcers, and heart problems.

Being negative can wear down your immune system. Ultimately, you will grow old to be the kind of person who people will stay away from.

Aside from being grumpy, you'll also have a lot of health issues to deal with.

Doctors found elevated levels of cortisol with people continually suffering from stress.

Anti-Age This Way Not That Way

This is a hormone associated with many of the degenerative diseases of aging.

When you let yourself get easily bothered with even the smallest things, you may as well say hello to hypertension, diabetes, obesity, and arthritis.

If you find that being positive is a little too difficult, there are things you can do.

Of course, it helps to talk to an expert, to someone who can help you cope with your problems.

Never take your body for granted. Make your doctor your friend. This is an indispensable method to prevent problems from burgeoning.

Then, you must realize the importance of having loved ones to stand by you when you see a storm brewing up.

Social relationships are not only fun, they're also very necessary to keep your mental health in check. The comfort of those who love you can help lessen your worries and ease your burdens.

They will give you a chance to air out your deepest concerns, and sometimes that could even be enough to make you feel better.

Always know that you have help available. Look within yourself and become more spiritual.

Believing in a higher power makes you realize that there is always someone out there looking out for you.

Everyone deserves to be happy. Just because fate hasn't dealt you the right cards yet does not mean you should lose hope.

As you grow older, you must take care of yourself more.

A good way to age gracefully is to know that life still has a few surprises up its sleeve.

When you wake up each day with renewed vigor, you'll soon realize that life can be good after all.

CHAPTER TEN

FASTING

Intermittent fasting
For decades doctors stressed the importance of taking breakfast and how that is the most important meal compared to lunch and dinner, but that science is challenged by new studies.

You know science progress by discovering the new, and the old is no longer the Holy Grail.

When I saw doctors on TV advocating the huge benefits of fasting, I knew we were at a new threshold.

The connection between fasting and anti-aging benefits started as an observatory experiment.

It appears that people who fast as a lifestyle especially for religious reasons appear to age slower than those who don't.

Why is fasting assisting in the anti-aging process we know that certain outcomes happen because of fasting for example the oldest man to ever run a marathon being over 100 years old he fasted basically for his entire life and he can run a full marathon not walk the marathon … but actually run the marathon as a 100 plus year old man

You would like to know the biological secret that can get you to a level where you can run a marathon at 100 years old?

Is there something to fasting?
Several scientist decided to get deeper into that.

They want to find out if there is any basis for that, something behind the scene that makes that a fact.

They worked with different living organism, since they want to understand what's happening at the cellular level

They worked with nematodes, rats etc. these subjects are easier to study before investigating humans.

One study found out that restricted intake of calories for nematodes extended their lifespan.

The reason for that increase was due to mitochondria growth mitochondria as you know is the powerhouse of the cell.

This mitochondria growth is stimulated by the increased production of an enzyme called AMPK or AMP Kinase when the cell discovered low energy due to less calorie

It was discovered that rats exposed to intermittent fasting were less likely to come down with the ailments found in rats not subjected to that.

There has been some debates if fasting really works or its just calorie intake restriction?

Anti-Age This Way Not That Way

There was a study done between two groups, both groups took the same amount of calories, the only thing that was different was that one group took breakfast, lunch and dinner while the other group will undergone intermittent fasting.

The result shows that the group that engaged in intermittent fasting had increased health markers

But there was one more study that took this research to another level

A study led by Dr. Ming Wiesel conducted at the Georgia State University in Atlanta realized that there was a specific molecule that prevents vascular aging and preventing vascular aging is really important because that can assist in preventing Alzheimer's, cardiovascular and cancer diseases that are related specifically to the fact that you are aging

These aforementioned diseases are associated with old age, your body starts to deteriorate specifically in the vascular area and this molecule is beta-hydroxyl butyrate, this is a ketone that is developed in the liver when your body has to switch from using glucose as energy to using ketones as energy now

During a 24 hour fast for example, a person will be getting their primary energy from beta-hydroxybutyrate, you can aim for 16 hour fast, where you eat your entire day's meal within 8 hours period, 16/8 formula.

Another way to get the benefits of beta-hydroxybutyrate is if you exercise while fasting you deplete your glucose energy level very quickly and then even though you're fasting for shorter than 24 hours, you'll be in the range of utilizing beta-hydroxybutyrate

Beta-hydroxybutyrate is a ketone that helps mobilize and burn fat. Your body starts to use that as your primary source of energy because you have no glucose, so we know that it helps in inducing anti-aging

Beta-hydroxybutyrate actually triggers a chain reaction in the body, where the DNA actually keeps the endothelial cells young and undamaged by simply bouncing off the beta-hydroxybutyrate that's being excreted in your body.

When the beta-hydroxybutyrate triggers the DNA in the endothelial cells it then attaches to an RNA binding protein which then boosts the activity of a stem cells transcriptional factor called Oct 4.

OCT 4 then increases Lamin b1 a key factor against DNA damaged, which then keeps the blood vessels young, because of that entire chain reaction from the fact that you were fasting you are now much less likely to have cardiovascular diseases.

Studies like this are not simply giving you just the biomarkers in participants that partook in fasting, it's showing you the actual biological process of why anti-

Anti-Age This Way Not That Way

aging is occurring in the body because of the molecule beta-hydroxylbutyrate.

Thanks for reading. Knowledge won't do any good unless there is action. Knowledge demands responsibility.

About the author

Kristine Knutson is a family therapist that lives in the United States. She is passionate in helping people enjoy healthy and meaningful lives. She is excited to contribute her knowledge and expertise so people can live the best life possible.

Her books present evidence-based principles in a ready-to-apply format, so people can lose weight, look younger, give up addictions, overcome toxic emotions, gain genuine confidence, fight off and prevent disease among others.

You can send her a mail, drkristineknutson@gmail.com

Other titles by the author include:

Lose weight This Way Not That Way:
Lose weight without dieting, even while you sleep and keep it off forever

Break Bad Habits This Way Not That Way:
Quit any addiction, break any habit without will power

Girl – Get Self Confidence This Way Not That Way:
Dissolve All Self-Doubts, Body Dissatisfaction, Appearance Anxiety. Enjoy Infinite Self-Worth and Magnetic Self-confidence.

Men – Get Self Confidence This Way Not That Way:
Find Your Infinite Self-Worth, Find Self Control and Demonstrate Self Confidence That Never Fails.

Anti-Age This Way Not That Way:
A science-based anti-aging plan that remarkably slow down and reverse your age.

www.ingramcontent.com/pod-product-compliance
Lightning Source LLC
Chambersburg PA
CBHW031410250726
48656CB00002B/612